TIPS FOR SUCCESSFUL EXCLUSIVE BREASTFEEDING

OVERCOMING COMMON CHALLENGES OF EXCLUSIVE BREASTFEEDING

CHERRY JOE

Disclaimer: The author's views and opinions are those of the book, not necessarily the official position or policy of any institution or organization. The author and publisher are not responsible for any losses or damages resulting from the use of or reliance on the offered content; the information is only provided for educational and informational reasons. Before making any decisions based on the information in this book, readers are urged to consult professionals and do their own research

TABLE OF CONTENTS

Introduction

Due to its effect on morbidity and mortality, particularly in young children under 1 year old, breastfeeding is a crucial component of a child's nutritional development and has significant consequences for the welfare of human health. Therefore, the importance of choosing breast milk as a food during the first six months of life is widely agreed upon by organizations devoted to the health of infants, and it is regarded as a vital public health policy. The WHO is a global health organization supports starting breastfeeding as soon as possible after birth and breastfeeding exclusively throughout the first six months of a child's life. The WHO has established the 2025 Global Nutrition

Targets, which are intended to enhance nutrition for pregnant women, infants, and young children. The sixth aim among them has breastfeeding as a priority: "increase the rate of exclusive breastfeeding in the first 6 months up to at least 50%.

Breastfeeding is cited by the United Nations Children's Fund (UNICEF) as a significant indication, saying that "Breastmilk alone is the perfect food for all infants in the first six months of life." Exclusive breastfeeding not only provides the best nutrition for infants but also boosts their immune systems and reduces their risk of passing away from acute respiratory illnesses and diarrhea. Additionally, it guards against long-term illnesses including diabetes and obesity [3]. However, UNICEF recently reported that despite the evidence supporting its short- and long-term effects, such as a protective role against childhood infections, an increase in intelligence, and a lower prevalence of diabetes and being overweight [4], many countries still underestimate the advantages of breastfeeding.

Additionally, the American Academy of Pediatrics has reiterated its advice to breastfeed exclusively for about 6 months before continuing to do so as complementary foods are introduced for at least a year, if both the mother and the child so desire [5]. Rare medical conditions are considered to be contraindications to breastfeeding. Furthermore, in their previous policy statement on breastfeeding, they acknowledged that the choice to breastfeed should not be seen by the mother, the doctor, or society as a lifestyle option but rather as a fundamental and important health choice that affects the welfare of the baby and the mother and should, therefore, be taken into consideration regardless of the parenting style or as a straightforward nutritional issue.It was underlined that in order for professionals to truly support and advocate for breastfeeding, they needed to look beyond the maternal-infant dyad and incorporate new ideas into their routines.

A high level of protection, promotion, and support for breastfeeding is thought to have the potential to avert 1.3 million child deaths annually [8]. Breastfeeding is also connected with a considerable reduction in infant mortality and morbidity in lower income nations. It has been calculated that 56.4% of hospital admissions for infections of non perinatal origin may be avoided if infants under 1 year old were breastfed for at least 4 months [9]. Additionally, there is proof that breastfeeding reduces the frequency and severity of atopic illnesses, digestive, respiratory, urinary, and middle ear infections, as well as sepsis and necrotizing enterocolitis in children. Breastfeeding has positive long-term impacts on cardiovascular risk factors, lowers the likelihood of childhood obesity, and enhances cognitive development. In addition, compared to women who have never breastfed, breastfeeding mothers had a lower risk of breast cancer, better birth spacing, and diabetes and ovarian cancer.

Chapter 1: Exclusive Breastfeeding, what is it?

The term "exclusive breastfeeding" refers to feeding newborns exclusively breast milk, whether it is expressed or taken directly from the breast, with the exception of drops or syrups containing vitamins, minerals, or other medications. One of the most important things for a baby's survival and development is exclusive breastfeeding. Due to its many advantages for both mother and child, it's also among the best gifts a new mother can give both her child and herself. Like arming, exclusive breastfeeding

Breastfeeding is still the simplest, healthiest, and least expensive feeding option that meets the needs of almost all newborns. Even though there is ample evidence to promote exclusive breastfeeding for the first six months of life, this practice is still not often practiced. There has been a lot of debate about exclusive breastfeeding, especially among first-time mothers. One debate topic is whether a youngster can only be fed breast milk to satisfy their hunger.

2. Just how much milk can a mother produce?

3. Given that water is so vital to human existence, why would a mother deprive her child of it?

and countless additional inquiries

This book will give a mother all the information and support she needs to embark on the pleasant adventure of exclusive breastfeeding.

Chapter 2: benefits of Exclusive Breastfeeding

It is impossible to overstate the value of exclusive breastfeeding. It lessens the risks of illnesses and infections. Additionally, mothers are thought to benefit from it as well.
The benefits of exclusive breastfeeding for children include:

1. Optimal Nutrition: Breast milk is regarded as the best nourishment for infants as it contains all the vitamins, minerals, and other nutrients required for healthy growth and development. Additionally, because it digests efficiently, there is a lower chance of

experiencing digestive issues like constipation and diarrhea.

2. Stronger Immune System: Antibodies in breast milk help protect babies from infections and illnesses like diarrhea, respiratory infections, and ear infections. Sudden Infant Death Syndrome (SIDS) and the risk of allergies, asthma, and eczema have also been linked to exclusive breastfeeding.

3.Cognitive Development: Research has found that breastfed infants have higher memory and learning skills as well as greater cognitive development. This might be because breast milk contains long-chain polyunsaturated fatty acids (LCPs), which are crucial for brain development.

5. Bonding: Breastfeeding encourages mother-child bonds since it involves cuddling and skin-to-skin contact. This encourages emotions like love, warmth, and stability, all of which are crucial for a child's emotional growth.

5. Lower Risk of Obesity: Babies who are breastfed have a lower chance of growing up to be overweight or obese. This is due to the fact that breast milk has the ideal ratio of nutrients to calories, which helps control desire and discourage overeating.

6. Lower Risk of Obesity: Babies who are breastfed have a lower chance of growing up to be overweight or obese. This is due to the fact that breast milk has the ideal ratio of nutrients to calories, which helps control desire and discourage overeating.

7. Economical: Exclusive breastfeeding is an economical strategy to ensure that newborns receive the best nutrition possible. Breast milk can save parents money and time because it is free and doesn't need to be prepared or sterilized like infant formula does.

Advantages for mothers of exclusively breastfeeding

1. Reduced Risk of Breast and Ovarian Cancer: A mother's risk of breast and ovarian cancer can be decreased by exclusively breastfeeding. The longer a mother breastfeeds her child, the greater the protective benefit, according to study.

2. Quicker Postpartum Recovery: The uterus grows back to its pre-pregnancy size more quickly thanks to the hormone

oxytocin, which is released during breastfeeding. This can lessen postpartum bleeding and aid in women' quicker postpartum recovery.

3. Exclusive breastfeeding saves money because it eliminates the need for formula, bottles, or sterilization supplies, making it an economical method of feeding a newborn.

4. Convenient: Breastfeeding is a convenient and time-saving method of feeding a baby because mothers may do it whenever and wherever they choose without having to make any special preparations.

5. Emotional Bonding: Breastfeeding can help a woman and her infant form a close emotional attachment. During breastfeeding, skin-to-skin contact

produces hormones that encourage maternal

bonding and make the mother feel closer to her child.

Chapter 3: how to increase milk supply in breast.

Concern over how breast milk alone may satiate a baby's hunger is one of the factors that prevents some mothers from starting exclusive breastfeeding for their children.
. You will be able to respond to this as a mother or a midwife if you have sufficient knowledge of breast milk and its supply. We will outline a few techniques for increasing breast milk supply in this chapter.

Breast milk Booster Foods.

Certainly! The following foods have a reputation for increasing the production of breast milk:

1. Oats: Oats are a good source of iron, fiber, and a soluble fiber that lowers cholesterol. The hormone prolactin, which is in charge of milk production, is also known to rise in response to them.

2. Fenugreek: For ages, women have utilized this plant to produce more breast milk. It is rich in iron, calcium, and other minerals and includes phytoestrogens that can increase milk production.

3.Fennel: Another herb that has been used for ages to boost milk production is fennel. It has a lot of vitamin C, calcium, and other minerals, as well as phytoestrogens that can increase milk production.

4. Spinach: A fantastic source of folic acid, iron, and calcium, spinach is also a great food for nursing women.

Additionally, it contains a lot of phytoestrogens, which may aid in raising milk production.

5.Almonds: Almonds are an excellent source of fiber, protein, and beneficial fats. Additionally, they have calcium and other essential minerals for nursing mothers.

6. Carrots: The beta-carotene found in carrots can be transformed by the by the body into Vitamin A. Both the mother and the child immune system needs Vitamin A to develop into a healthy adult.

7. Nuts: Packed with antioxidants and good lipids, nuts can improve the taste of milk. Walnuts, almonds, cashew and pistachios
Raw or roasted almonds make a good snack if your milk supply is low. Toss

them into salads, smoothies, cookies, or just snack on them in between meals.

8. Brewer's Yeast: Brewer's yeast is another natural lactation help. Large amounts of chromium, selenium, iron, and B vitamins are included in this superfood. Your body requires these nutrients to produce the most milk possible while nursing.
You can consume brewer's yeast as a supplement or cook it into food, depending on your tastes. It pairs well with sweets like homemade muffins and pancakes.

9.Seeds: Flaxseeds, pumpkin seeds, and sesame seeds are all nutritious additions to your diet. These meals are loaded with beneficial fats and minerals that support your body's ability to create milk.

They can be added to smoothies, added to salads, or eaten as a snack.

10. Asparagus: Asparagus possesses what are referred to as "estrogenic properties" that increase prolactin levels in the body and increase milk production. Due to its galactagogue (an herb that helps to promote the production of breastmilk) qualities, this vegetable has been utilized in Ayurvedic medicine for a very long time.
It aids in boosting and maintaining milk secretion since it is high in flavonoids and saponins. It promotes reproductive health while also easing stomach problems.

11.Milk Thistle: This plant has estrogen-stimulating effects. Regular consumption raises prolactin levels and boosts breast milk production. You can consume milk thistle as a supplement or in teas. Salads, curries, and vegetable dishes all benefit from its seeds.

12. Green papayas: This exotic fruit is loaded with enzymes and phytochemicals that promote milk production and breast health. Additionally, it provides modest sedative properties that aid in relaxation.

Dedicated Breastfeeding Practices that Benefit Mothers

1. Keeping hydrated by consuming lots of fluids, especially water.

2. Consuming a diet rich in fruits, vegetables, whole grains, and lean proteins that is well-balanced and healthy.

3. Getting as much rest as you can, including naps while the baby is napping.

4. Refrain from using tobacco products, alcohol, or caffeine as they can harm the unborn child and affect milk production.

5. Maintaining a breastfeeding schedule and nursing often to assist the infant acquire enough nutrition and sustain the milk supply.

6. Possibilities for breastfeeding that are cozy and encouraging, as well as a welcoming environment for nursing.

7. Burping the infant after feedings will help to avoid colic and gas.

8. Seeking assistance from a healthcare professional or lactation consultant if you are having pain or trouble nursing.

9. Practicing good personal hygiene, such as cleaning hands and breasts before feeding, to avoid infections.

10. Continuing to have a happy and carefree attitude toward breastfeeding in order to lessen stress and foster a bond with the infant.

Additionally, you should be aware that the first few weeks won't be easy and that the baby will suck longer and more frequently. Don't be disheartened, though; this is quite normal and the infant will start to adjust with time. In the process of exclusively breastfeed

Chapter 4: Breastfeeding Exclusively while working as a mother.

It can be challenging for working-class mothers to balance the obligations of employment with breastfeeding. It takes a lot of work, dedication, and preparation to ensure that your child is fed properly while maintaining your work schedule. We will go through a few strategies for working-class mothers to manage exclusive breastfeeding in this article.

1. Begin Early

While still pregnant, you must begin making preparations for exclusive breastfeeding. Go to prenatal classes and learn how to nurse effectively. Start extracting breast milk and freezing it as well. When you're away from your infant, having a large supply of frozen breast milk can be useful.

2. Establish a feeding routine
Establish a feeding plan that is convenient for you and your infant. Establishing a schedule for your baby's feedings is essential so that you can organize your workday around it. By doing so, you may better manage your time while making sure your baby receives the necessary amount of milk. If you have a supportive partner or family member, they can assist by watching the baby while it feeds, allowing you to concentrate on your work.

3.Utilize a breast pump.
For mothers in the working class, a breast pump is a fantastic tool. You can extract milk and save it for a later time. Even when you're not with your baby, you can still give them breast milk by using a breast pump. During your lunch

break or any other break you get at work, you can express milk.

4. Consult with your boss

Inform your employer about your breastfeeding requirements. The majority of companies support breastfeeding mothers and are prepared to aid them by making reasonable arrangements. Talk about choices like having a private area to pump in or having a flexible work schedule that enables you to take breaks for breastfeeding or pumping.

5. Prepare your nursing supplies

Bring along all the equipment you'll need for breastfeeding, such as a breast pump, milk storage containers or bags, nipple cream, nursing pads, and a nursing cover or scarf. It may be simpler to pump or breastfeed while working or traveling if you have all your breastfeeding materials in one location.

6. Seek assistance

For working-class moms in particular, breastfeeding can be difficult. Ask other mothers who have experienced the same thing for support. Join a support group for breastfeeding or go to a lactation consultant's sessions. They can assist you stay exclusively breastfeeding by providing guidance and encouragement.

7. Look for yourself

It's crucial to look after yourself when nursing. Get enough sleep, eat a diet that is balanced, and drink lots of water. Taking care of oneself is essential to prevent burnout because breastfeeding may be physically and emotionally taxing.

In conclusion, working-class moms may find it difficult to exclusively breastfeed, but it is feasible to do so with commitment, preparation, and support. Don't forget to get a head start, plan your feedings, utilize a breast pump, speak with your employer, pack your nursing equipment, get support, and look after yourself. With the help of these suggestions, you can continue to be a productive working mother while giving your infant the nourishment they need.

Chapter 5: tips for Exclusive C-section Breastfeeding

1. For all neonates, including those delivered by cesarean section (C-section), exclusive nursing is advised. While exclusive breastfeeding may present some difficulties for C-section women, there are a number of solutions:

2. Begin nursing as soon as you can: Even if it is challenging or uncomfortable because of pain and discomfort from the C-section, it is crucial to begin breastfeeding as soon as you can following delivery. By ensuring the infant obtains colostrum, which is rich in nutrients and antibodies, this can help build a milk supply.

3. Select a cozy position: The secret to successful breastfeeding is to select a cozy nursing position Try out various

holds, including the cradle hold or the football hold, to see which one is most comfortable for you and your infant.

4. Take pain relievers: Breastfeeding may be challenging for C-section mothers who endure pain and discomfort. To reduce pain and make it easier for you to breastfeed, it's crucial to take prescribed painkillers as prescribed.

5. Use a nursing pillow: While breastfeeding, a nursing cushion can support the infant and ease pressure on the incision area.

6. Seek assistance: Speak with a lactation specialist or a breastfeeding support group for assistance. They can offer advise and ideas that will make nursing more convenient and comfortable.

7. Exercise patience: Exclusive breastfeeding can be challenging, so it's crucial to be persistent and patient. Never give up and always ask for assistance.

Overall, C-section women can successfully breastfeed exclusively with the correct encouragement and support. Prioritize breastfeeding and ask for assistance when necessary.

Conclusion.

Exclusive breastfeeding is the practice of supplying a baby for the first six months of life with nothing but breast milk. It is regarded as the best approach to feed a baby throughout the first six months of life and offers major health advantages to both the mother and the child. The advantages of exclusive breastfeeding and the justifications for its promotion have been covered in this essay.

The nutritious value of breast milk is one of the most significant advantages of exclusive breastfeeding. Protein, lipids, and vitamins included in breast milk are vital for the development and maintenance of growing babies. Additionally, it contains antibodies that help shield infants from illnesses and infections. Infants are less prone to suffer from digestive issues like constipation or diarrhea since breast milk is easily absorbed.

The mother-baby bonding experience is a significant advantage of exclusive breastfeeding. No other form of feeding can compare to the unique link that breastfeeding forges between mother and child. The physical proximity of nursing gives the baby comfort and security, while the process of breastfeeding causes the mother to release hormones that encourage relaxation and a sense of well-being.

For the woman, exclusively nursing provides tremendous health advantages. It lowers the risk of osteoporosis and breast and ovarian cancer in later life. Additionally, breastfeeding reduces

postpartum hemorrhage and benefits
both mother and child health globally.